11/10

Taking Care Of Myself

I Have DOWN Syndrome

Jenny Bryan

Gareth Stevens
Publishing

Please visit our Web site, www.garethstevens.com.
For a free color catalog of all our high-quality books,
call toll free 1-800-542-2595 or fax 1-877-542-2596.

Library of Congress Cataloging-in-Publication Data

Bryan, Jenny.
I have Down syndrome / Jenny Bryan.
    p. cm. — (Taking care of myself)
Includes index.
ISBN 978-1-4339-3857-3 (library binding)
1. Down syndrome—Popular works. I. Title.
RJ506.D68B79 2011
618.92'858842—dc22

                              2010014795

This edition first published in 2011 by
Gareth Stevens Publishing
111 East 14th Street, Suite 349
New York, NY 10003

Editorial Director: Kerri O'Donnell
Design Director: Haley Harasymiw

Photo Credits:
Wayland Publishers Ltd would like to thank: Moodboard/Alamy cover; Chapel Studios 26; The Down
Syndrome Association 9 (bottom), 22, 23, 24 (both); Angela Hampton, Family Life Picture Library 5, 7
(both), 18; Impact 25; Sally Lewis-Smith 29; The Riding for the Disabled Association 28; L. Willatt, East
Anglian Regional Genetics Service/Science Photo Library 6 (both), Hattie Young/Science Photo Library 8, 9.
All the other photographs were taken for Wayland by Angela Hampton. Most of the people who are
photographed in this book are models.

Printed in the China
CPSIA compliance information: Batch #WAS10GS: For further information contact Gareth Stevens, New York, New York at 1-800-542-2595.

Contents

Meet Stacey, Richie, Maria, and Jack

Stacey has Down syndrome. Every morning, she and her older sister, Jo, walk to their school, down the street from where they live. Stacey needs extra help with her reading and writing, but not with her favorite lesson, art. She often draws pictures of the family pets, especially their dog, Sammy.

▼ *After school, Megan often takes Richie to the playground or to the local swimming pool.*

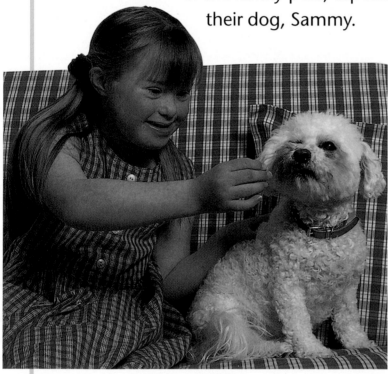

▲ *Stacey loves playing with Sammy and taking him out for long walks.*

Richie is five years old and he has Down syndrome, too. He loves playing with his big sister, Megan. When Mom and Dad first brought Richie home from the hospital, they were very worried about him, but Megan thought the new baby was great. Now, none of them can imagine life without Richie.

◄ *Maria and her roommates enjoy a cup of tea and a chat at the end of the day.*

Maria is 22 years old and she shares an apartment with three other young women—Sandy, Tina, and Rachel. They all have learning difficulties, Sandy is deaf, and Maria has Down syndrome. The four roommates do their own shopping and look after themselves, with a little help from Liz and Jim who live next door. Maria has a job at the local library.

Jack catches a bus each morning to take him to a special school for children with learning difficulties. The school is in another town, and the trip takes about an hour. Jack likes the other children at the school, but they don't live near him so he can only see them at school. He wishes he could go to the same school as his brother, Ben, so that he could make friends who live closer to home.

▲ *Jack's reading has gotten much better and he often reads to his brother, Ben.*

5

What Is Down Syndrome?

If you have Down syndrome, you have an extra chromosome in each of your cells. Chromosomes carry all the information we inherit from our parents, which affects how we look, grow, and feel.

Humans usually have 23 pairs of chromosomes, but people with Down syndrome have an extra copy of one chromosome. It doesn't sound like much of a difference. But that extra chromosome affects how the body and mind develop. That's why people like Stacey, Richie, Maria, and Jack may take longer than other children to learn to walk, speak, read, and write.

▼ *The chromosomes on the right are those of a person with Down syndrome, showing three chromosomes in the twenty-first set.*

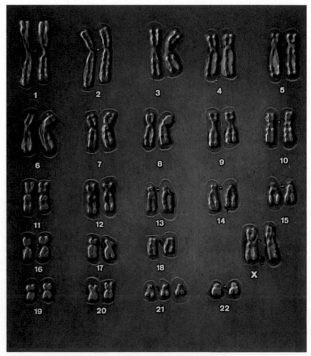

▼ *Babies with Down syndrome need a lot of care and attention, just like other babies.*

At birth, babies with Down syndrome tend to be small and their muscles may be weak. People with Down syndrome are also more likely to have heart defects, and many have problems with their eyesight or hearing. They also tend to have skin problems and may have a lot of coughs and colds, so they need to take extra care of themselves.

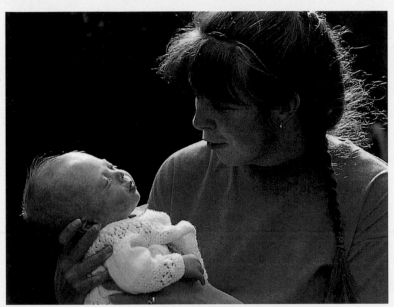

One in every 1,000 babies is born with Down syndrome. It happens all over the world. Women of all ages can have babies with Down syndrome, but it is more likely if a woman has a baby when she is in her late thirties or forties.

▶ *Toddlers learn quickly, especially if they have plenty of attention and help.*

7

Treatment for Down Syndrome

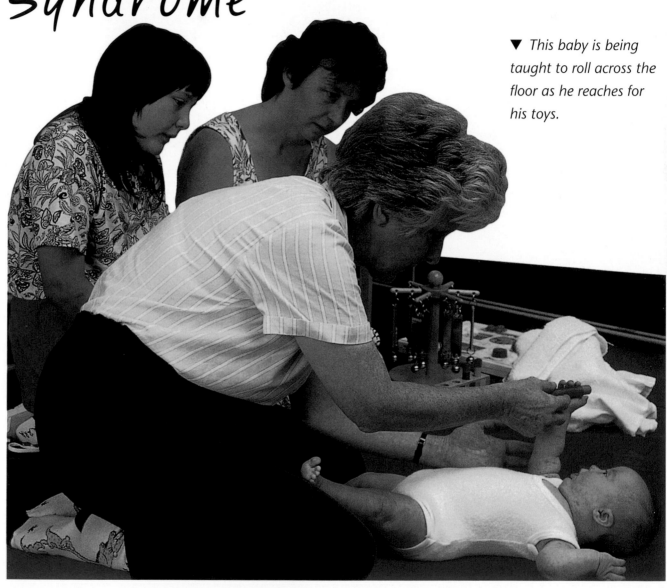

▼ *This baby is being taught to roll across the floor as he reaches for his toys.*

Doctors cannot take away the extra chromosome that people with Down syndrome have. But they can treat many of the health problems that may occur.

Children can have operations to correct heart problems. Wearing glasses or hearing aids can help to improve their eyesight and hearing. They may also need to do special exercises to make their muscles stronger, or have help to improve how they speak.

As they get older, people with Down syndrome tend to put on weight easily. They have to be careful not to eat too much and to get plenty of exercise to stay fit and healthy. Since people with Down syndrome may have a lot of coughs and colds, they sometimes need medicine to help them get better.

▲ *This boy has poor hearing so his mother is teaching him to use sign language to talk to her.*

Like Stacey and Jack, children with Down syndrome may need extra help with their lessons at school. Adults like Maria can get support and advice about finding jobs and their own places to live. They may also need someone to help them with things such as shopping and cooking, and to make sure they are taking good care of themselves.

◄ *Everyone needs skills to find a job. This man trained to use computers, which helped him get a job.*

Stacey's Day

◄ In math classes, Miss Jackson is on hand to help Stacey with difficult work.

▼ Art is one of Stacey's favorite subjects at school.

Stacey goes to the same lessons as other children at her school. But she and a boy in her class get a little extra help from Miss Jackson, the teacher's assistant. Miss Jackson sits with them during some lessons, such as math and science, and explains things they find hard to understand. Then they do the schoolwork just like the rest of the class.

In art, drama, and PE lessons, Stacey joins in with the other children and doesn't need Miss Jackson's help. Stacey has a part in the school play and she's helping to paint the scenery, too.

Stacey likes some sports more than others. She doesn't like ballgames. She tries very hard but she keeps dropping the ball. Some of the children laugh at her and they don't want her in their team. This makes Stacey feel sad.

"I really enjoy our swimming lessons at school. I like being in the water, and my friends and I usually end up splashing each other!"

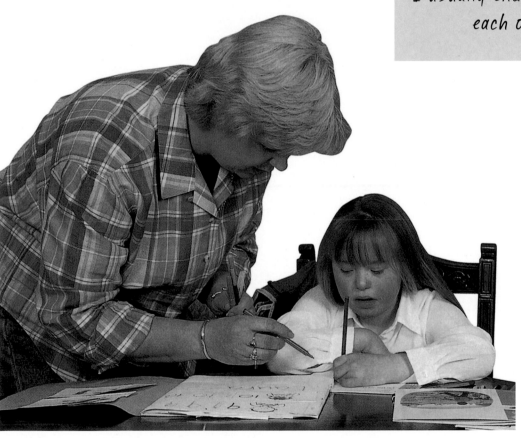

◄ *Mom makes sure Stacey does her homework and helps out if Stacey gets stuck.*

When she gets home from school, Stacey does her homework. Sometimes she bribes her sister with chocolate so that she will help her. Like her friends, Stacey would prefer to listen to her CDs than do homework, but her Mom can be very strict about homework!

Jack's Day

◀ *Jack answers lots of questions in class.*

Jack's Special Talent

"Woodwork is my favorite subject. I love the feel of smooth, polished wood. I feel really happy when I have finished making something."

Jack goes to a special school where all the pupils have learning difficulties. Some have Down syndrome, like Jack.

The lessons at Jack's school are the same as at other schools, but the teachers explain things more slowly, so that all the children understand. Jack finds math somewhat difficult but he enjoys history and geography.

◀ Jack's teacher is showing him how to use a saw safely.

▼ At recess, Jack and his friends rush outside for a game of soccer.

Jack also likes woodwork classes. Last semester, he made a spice rack for his mom. At home, Jack's grandpa makes lots of things in his workshop and Jack loves to help. When he grows up, Jack wants to make furniture.

Like Stacey, Jack isn't very good at ballgames, but neither are most of the other children in his class, so no one cares and they all have fun. People don't laugh at Jack when he drops the ball, and he doesn't feel left out.

Jack feels tired after the long bus ride home from school. He doesn't know the other children in his street. They all go to the local school and seem to have their own friends, so Jack feels a little lonely. He usually watches TV in the evening with Ben and their mom, but sometimes Mom takes Ben and Jack for a bike ride or to the movies.

Richie Faces the Bullies

Richie and Megan often take their dog, Bonny, for a walk in the park near their home. One day, they were throwing a ball for Bonny when some boys came over and started laughing at Richie.

▼ *Richie, Megan, and Bonny were having a great time until the bullies came along and spoiled it.*

"You look funny, your face is all flat," they said to Richie.

"Stupid, stupid!" they jeered. One of the boys shoved Richie and then his glasses fell off.

"Leave us alone," shouted Megan. But the boys grabbed the ball and ran away.

Megan was very upset. She hates it when people are unkind to Richie. But Richie said it didn't matter. He picked up his glasses and put them on. He began to make funny faces at Megan and soon they were both laughing.

"Now, you really do look funny," said Megan, and they started to throw sticks for Bonny to fetch.

Richie Doesn't Care!

"I don't get upset when people are nasty to me. I wouldn't want to be friends with them anyway!"

▶ Richie soon forgot the bullies and cheered up Megan.

Maria's Day

Maria found it hard to get a job. Most people did not want to give her work when they saw she had Down syndrome. They thought she couldn't do the job. She applied for jobs in stores and at a movie theater, but she didn't get them. She kept trying until she got a job at the library. Maria enjoys earning her own money to spend how she likes.

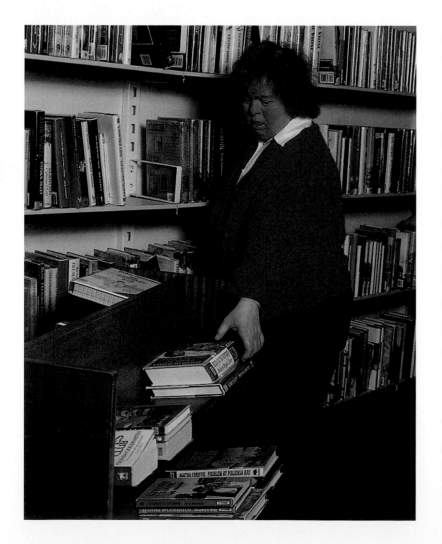

At the library, there is a cart full of books that people have read and brought back. Maria puts the books back on the shelves. There are many sections in the library, and Maria has to check each book to see where it belongs. Every book has a number on it and Maria has to put the books in the right order on the shelves.

◄ At the library, they gave Maria the chance to prove she could do the job, and she showed them that she could.

Sometimes Maria looks at the books before she puts them back. Once, when she was in the children's section of the library, a little girl asked Maria about the book she was reading. Maria started to tell her all about it, and the little girl liked the story. Her mother listened, too, and then she asked Maria about some other books. Now, Maria often helps the children to choose books.

Maria Loves Her Job

"I enjoy helping people to choose books from the library because I love reading myself. There are so many books to choose from."

▼ *When you're looking for a good book, it helps to get advice from someone who has read them.*

Growing Up

How old were you when your parents first let you go somewhere without them? Maybe it was just a walk to the store or to ride a bike or catch a bus to school. Or perhaps you started going to a friend's house to play or do your homework.

No one wants their parents around all the time when they are growing up, and parents like to spend some time on their own, too.

As you grow up, you'll spend more and more time doing what you want to do. You'll choose where to go and what to do, instead of leaving it up to your parents or other adults to decide. Sometimes you'll have a good time, sometimes you won't. But at least you can decide for yourself.

◄ *Children with Down syndrome have hobbies, just like everyone else.*

▶ *These girls love singing along to their favorite bands.*

When you leave school, you may go away to college or decide to live with some friends. It's an exciting time because you'll be in charge of your life. If you want to stay in bed all day, you can. If you want to stay up late watching TV, no one will tell you off.

▼ *It is good to have a friend to talk to.*

If you have learning difficulties, you will also want to make your own decisions. You will want to be as independent as possible. With a little help, you can live like other adults. Like Maria, you may be able to live where there are people who will help out if there is a problem, but will not interfere.

Maria's Outing

Maria wanted to go to the theater, but she needed someone to tell her how to get there. If you were giving her instructions, you would need to explain things very clearly. She isn't deaf, so you wouldn't need to shout. But you could help her by using easy words.

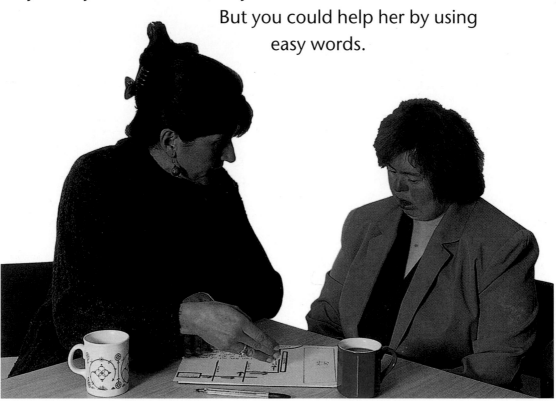

Maria asked Liz, who lives next door, to tell her how to get to the movie theater. Liz drew a simple map and told Maria to turn left out of her apartment, cross two big streets, and turn left, then right. Then she had to walk about 100 yards along the main road, past some stores and restaurants, until she reached the theater.

▲ To help Maria remember her route, Liz drew a map for Maria to take with her.

Liz suggested that Maria should watch for places she would pass on the way, like the mailbox on the corner, the big church, and the bus station.

When you are trying to remember something, it always helps to repeat what you have been told. So, before setting off, Maria described her route to her roommate, Tina.

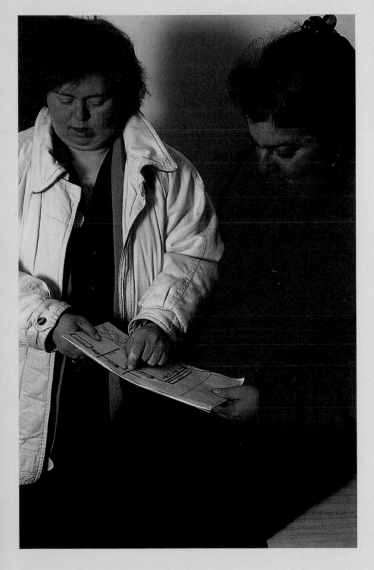

▲ Tina helped Maria to check that she understood how to find the movie theater.

▲ Liz's map was a big help and Maria wasn't nervous about finding the theater on her own.

With the help of Liz's map, Maria found the movie theater and enjoyed watching the movie. When she came out, it was raining, so she took the bus home. Liz had written down the name of the street where Maria would need to get off the bus. Maria showed it to the driver and he told her when they got there.

Everyone Is Different

Although they all have Down syndrome, Jack, Maria, Richie, and Stacey are very different from each other. They look different, they think differently, and they are good at different things. They all have an extra chromosome but they have inherited the information on their chromosomes from different parents. So they are as different from each other as you are from the other children in your class.

► *This baby girl will probably look like her mom when she's older, just as her brothers look like their father.*

People who have brown eyes don't all look the same, and neither do those with Down syndrome. Richie looks much more like his father than he looks like Jack. And, when she's a little older, Stacey will not look like Maria. She will look more like her mom.

◄ *Everyone is different. Life would be very boring if we were all the same!*

It's a mistake to think that people with the same problem with their health have the same abilities and disabilities. Just because two people are both blind, it doesn't mean they will be the same in other ways.

What do you do when you meet someone for the first time? You probably talk to them to find out about them. You are more likely to make friends with them if they are interested in the same things as you. Whether you have Down syndrome or not, you will only find out what someone is like if you get to know them. You can't guess what they are like just by looking at them.

Aiming High

▲ *Philip Lee and his partner have to do a lot of training to get fit for their charity bike rides.*

People with Down syndrome have done some great things.

Philip Lee has ridden his bicycle in Israel and Jordan, even cycling 300 miles (483 kilometers) through the desert to raise money for charity.

James Van Maggs, a successful musician and dancer, has taken part in many competitions and has won awards. Despite his busy life, he has even found time to learn to speak German.

Timmy Lang is an actor and has appeared on television. He was so good at remembering his lines that the other actors called him "One Take Tim," because they never had to film his part twice.

Tracey Young couldn't walk until she was five years old, but today she twirls around the dance floor and wins prizes for her Latin-American dancing.

▲ *To play the violin as well as James Van Maggs takes a great deal of practice.*

▲ *Athletes receiving medals at the Special Olympics.*

People with Down syndrome are among hundreds of athletes from all over the world who compete in the Special Olympics—a sports competition for people with learning and physical disabilities.

All over the world, people with Down syndrome have been successful, whether they have gotten the job they wanted, appeared in a play, won prizes in sports, or learned to play a musical instrument. Sometimes you have to struggle to get what you want, but if you have to work a little harder than most people, success feels even better.

If you aim high, you can do a lot with your life, whether you have learning difficulties or not. It may be tough and it may take longer than you expected, but if you want something enough, you can do it!

Making Life Easier

Whate changes would you make in the way we treat people with Down syndrome? How could we make it easier for them to do well in school, become independent, get a job, and take part in all the activities that we enjoy?

▼ Computers in schools can help people to learn different skills.

In the future, doctors may find ways to improve the eyesight and hearing of people with Down syndrome, and to treat their heart problems more easily. Perhaps they will also be able to help children with Down syndrome to fight off coughs, colds, and other infections more effectively.

The most important thing is to give everyone the chance to learn all they can, and to use their skills. If you are good at art, like Stacey, or woodwork, like Jack, you may be able to use those skills when you are older to get a job or just to enjoy yourself and have fun.

Some people with Down syndrome do better in ordinary schools, like the one Stacey goes to. Others prefer a special school, like Jack's. But if they don't get the chance to go to the school that suits them best, they may never do as well as they could. Parents want a wider choice of schools for children with Down syndrome.

If people with Down syndrome have the same opportunities as everyone else to train for a job or career, they can be reliable and good at their work, like Maria. With a little help, we can all live independently. In the future, perhaps we will.

◀ *Finding the right career is as important for people with Down syndrome as it is for other adults.*

Getting Help

None of the medical, educational, and other changes that you have just read about will make any difference to people with Down syndrome if we don't help them, too.

Everybody has felt sad or left out at some time. It isn't a very nice feeling. It is unkind and unfair to laugh, stare, or ignore somebody just because they look different. Like everyone else, they feel upset and lonely when people won't give them a chance.

Children with Down syndrome want to take part in the same activities as others of their age. They want to join clubs and groups.

◄ *Groups such as the Federation of Riding for the Disabled help people with disabilities to enjoy horse riding.*

▶ Lots of special schools, clubs, and organizations plan trips and activities especially for people with Down syndrome.

The National Down Syndrome Society (NDSS) provides educational advice and information about health issues, research, and events connected with Down syndrome. You can contact them via their telephone helpline at 1-800-221-4602 or email info@ndss.org. The telephone line is open Monday through Friday, 9–5 Eastern Standard Time, and offers support in 150 different languages.

The NDSS also has affiliates throughout the United States, which you can find by doing a search on their web site. You can also read and share inspiring success stories written by people with Down syndrome from all across the country.

Through this and similar organizations, people with Down syndrome and their families can get help and advice about everyday health, therapy, education, and practical problems, and they can discuss the solutions. These groups can also offer advice about training, housing, and leisure activities.

Glossary

Cells The smallest parts of any living thing. The human body is made up of millions of cells, which do many different jobs.

Chromosome A threadlike structure found in cells. It carries the genes (inherited information) that play a big part in deciding how a person looks and thinks and the way their body works.

Defects Things that have gone wrong or don't work properly.

Independent Able to look after yourself without relying on other people to help or to make decisions for you.

Infections Illnesses caused by tiny organisms.

Inherit To be born with physical and mental characteristics that have been physically passed on to you by your parents.

Learning difficulties Problems learning how to do things, such as math, reading, or writing. People with learning difficulties may take longer to learn new skills.

Roommates People who share a home, even though they are not usually from the same family.

Further Reading

Books to Read

Down Syndrome
by Angela Royston
Heinemann Library, 2005

Let's Talk About It: My Friend Has Down Syndrome
by Jennifer Moore-Mallinos
Barron's Educational Series, 2008

We Can Do It!
by Laura Dwight
Star Bright Books, 2005

Web Sites

http://kidshealth.org/kid/health_problems/birth_defect/down_syndrome.html

http://kids.nationalgeographic.com/Stories/PeoplePlaces/Downsyndrome

Index